JOSEPH CORVO'S
BACKACHE CURE

JOSEPH CORVO'S BACKACHE CURE

by

Joseph Corvo

VERMILION
LONDON

First published in 1992 by Vermilion
an imprint of Ebury Press
Random Century House
20 Vauxhall Bridge Road
London SW1V 2SA

A catalogue record for this book is available
from the British Library.

ISBN 0-09-175433-X

Photographs © Barnaby Hopkins
Design by Behram Kapadia
Typeset by 𝍣 Tek Art Ltd., Addiscombe, Croydon, Surrey.
Printed in England by Clays Ltd, St Ives plc

Contents

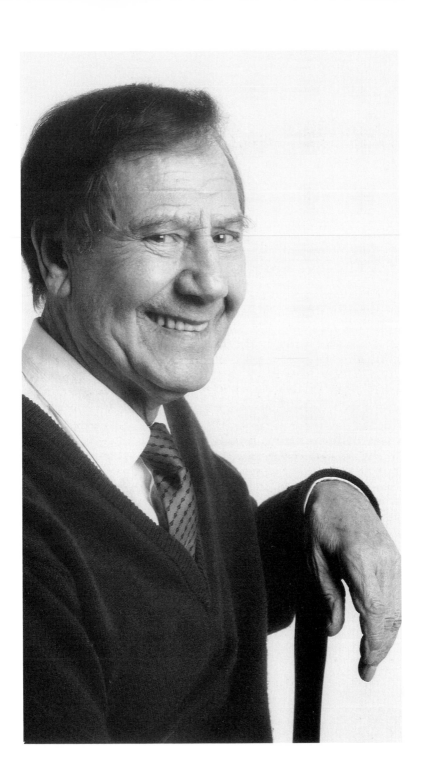

A Message from Joseph Corvo

Zone Therapy is a method of concentrating the body's own miraculous healing powers. You can treat yourself at home and obtain miraculous results in an amazingly short time. If you have the desire to succeed, you will succeed. Persist and Zone Therapy will keep you in perfect condition for the rest of your life.

This is the great secret of Zone Therapy. The electro-magnetic forces which animate your body run through it in ten major zones, feeding and regenerating all the glands and organs in those zones. Illness, ageing and pain occur when toxins accumulate at the nerve endings so that the flow of the electro-magnetic forces becomes blocked, thereby causing glands and organs to malfunction and wither. Zone Therapy is a unique system of pressure point massage which disperses these toxins so that the body's own animating and healing powers can course through the body at full force again.

Apart from the many famous and successful people who come to my clinic, including members of the royal family and show-business stars, countless people all over the world have now been converted to Zone Therapy through my bestselling books *Joseph Corvo's Zone Therapy, The Natural Facelift* and *Joesph Corvo's Instant Headache Cure*. Once people begin experiencing the benefits of Zone Therapy they never give up.

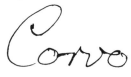

Introduction

Sixty per cent of people suffer from severe back pain between the ages of fifteen and thirty-six, and as we get older back pain is more and more likely to be a problem. For millions of people in the UK alone back pain is so bad that it seriously affects their lives. Moreover UK government statistics show that every year sixty million working days are lost through back trouble. The NHS spends over £350 million per year trying, mostly ineffectually, to treat back problems.

The good news is that by practising Zone Therapy for just half an hour every day you can cure almost all back problems. Many back problems can be cleared up completely in just one session. All but the most deep-seated can be cured in a matter of days. Persist and you need never suffer from back pain again.

One of the most common complaints among people who come to see me at my clinic is backache, and in my experience the application of Zone Therapy to backache shows this treatment at its most miraculous. I have asked some of my patients to write me testimonials for this book:

Dearest Joe

Just a quick line to say how much you have helped me over the years.

As you know I broke my back in 1986 and my back was broken in two places which resulted in devastating pain and a threat of permanent paralysis.

Straight out of intensive care I turned to you, dear Joe, and your Zone Therapy, and most definitely it was a major factor in the long, slow, healing process. Zone Therapy encouraged the spine to knit and the nerves to grow which had been severed. It also gave me the energy I needed to fight on as my body was being attacked on every front by bronchitis, kidney infections, and liver disorders.

It helped to draw out the residual shock form the body – the result of any major accident – and to tackle the problem of insomnia. A daily session of Zone Therapy was constructive in itself but also a vital boost to make me, the patient, feel I could help recovery in a positive way.

When lying in a hospital bed, being turned by five nurses every two hours, a light massage on the feet was the only thing to bring me relief from the burning pain.

And now, dear Joe, I am leading a normal life, able to walk, something that it seemed I would never do again.

I do my Zone Therapy every day to myself and I thank God and you all the time for the many blessings bestowed upon me. What great joy to be free from pain and anguish.

All my love always

Roz Hamburg

Dear Joe

I am writing to you to thank you for all you have done for me.

As you know when I saw you I had a seven-year history of severe back trouble which had confined me to bed for up to ten days at a time on an almost regular six-monthly basis.

Your treatment was nothing short of miraculous, miraculous.

I had been to orthopaedic surgeons, chiropractors, manipulative surgeons, physiotherapists, faith healers and anything or anyone else I could find as I looked for a cure or even a relief of my condition.

All offered either temporary relief through drugs or manipulation. But none offered me a permanent cure.

I recall your advice on my first visit to you: that if I did exactly as you advised I would never have back pain again. I found that hard to believe: everyone else had failed so what was so special about Zone Therapy? I was about to find out. Joe, you gave me six treatments and showed me what to do. You said it would take twelve sessions doing it to myself.

After the six treatments all pain and discomfort had disappeared. I simply could not believe it. I was cured. Unfortunately I deemed myself cured and I was for a period of *five years – trouble-free for five years.*

Then just recently my back trouble returned with a vengeance, and I had to call upon your powers again for your kind help.

You wagged a finger at me and said, 'Robert, you disobeyed the laws of cause and effect and have taken the risk of not completing the full treatment'.

It is now five weeks since I restarted the Zone Therapy and the pain and discomfort has completely gone. But this time I intend to give myself Zone Therapy for the rest of my life. I feel so good to be cured and out of pain, this time permanently.

Again I am amazed at your healing ability. You are someone very special. I know I owe my comfort in life over the past five years to you, Joe.

But I believe that your methods involve more than Zone Therapy. You have a divine healing gift which is reflected through your Christianity and pure godliness.

God bless you, Joseph, and thank you.

Yours very sincerely

ROBERT L NELSON *LLB*

Dear Joseph

After a year or more suffering terribly from a crippling sciatic nerve and hip condition and having made so many fruitless visits to physiotherapists, osteopaths etc, etc – no results – I at last discovered Zone Therapy.

You have succeeded totally in carrying out a truly miraculous cure and have left me absolutely confident that should I ever have any other complaints of this nature, you will be able to remedy them with your unique gifts and wonderful Zone Therapy. What a marvellous method of therapy treatment it is. Fantastic is the best way to describe it. Everyone should do it.

With renewed thanks always

ANNE BASSINGHERD MUNDY

Dear Joseph

I want to thank you and Zone Therapy. I suffered with chronic back trouble from the age of fourteen years old.

I visited all the doctors available as well as acupuncturists, chiropractors and all the other available treatments I could find. You name it, I tried it. All without success. I was told I would have to live with it. Can you imagine, because I was completely fit otherwise; a good skier, horse polo. I did all these things with continual back pain and the pain became part of me and my life.

Then I heard about you. How does one thank someone who performs a cure on them? You, Joe, completely cured my back after all those years of pain. I am now free from its bondage. I am lost for words. You possess something very special – of that there is absolutely no doubt.

Bless you, Joe, always.

EDWARD HUTLEY

What these people suffered from is very common because the back is one of the most delicate parts of the human body.

The human body has 214 bones, all of them living fibrous tissue and all of them connected in different ways to the spine. The spine also carries the central nervous system which controls and co-ordinates circulation, respiration, the digestive organs and the movement of limbs. The spine is particularly susceptible to injury, and any injury to the back will have very serious repercussions for the whole body; any injury to the spine immediately affects the nervous system, your muscles, your organs and your glands. You soon begin to feel run down and depressed.

The system of treatment that follows – unlike many other forms of treatment – involves no direct manipulation of the back which can be extremely dangerous. Also unlike other treatments it involves healing the nerves, muscles, organs and glands which are damaged by back injury.

Apply Zone Therapy's simple system with conviction and you will feel the body's own natural healing power flowing through you. Many of my patients call me a miracle man, but Joseph Corvo doesn't have to treat you personally in order for you to benefit from Zone Therapy's miraculous healing properties. Follow the simple instructions contained in the next chapter and you are going to feel better.

Joseph Corvo's Backache Cure

I am going to show you precisely which pressure points you need to massage in order to rid yourself of backache. Remember, the aim of this massage is to disperse toxins which have accumulated on your nerve endings and which are therefore blocking the free flow of your body's own miraculous healing powers. So you must rub as vigorously as possible – this is a practical, medical treatment, not something which is merely ethereal or occult. Positive thinking, and a determination to succeed, is vital to this treatment, but it is not by itself enough. You must massage the pressure points vigorously and for the lengths of time specified. Persist and you *will* rid yourself of backache.

If you use your fingers or your thumbs you may be able to feel the grit under your skin where the toxic crystals have accumulated. In order to disperse them as quickly as possible press as hard as you can bear. If your fingers and thumbs are not strong enough, use, for example, the top of a pencil with a rounded edge or a toothbrush handle. Whether you are using fingers, thumbs or a rounded instrument, you will find that any pressure points with blockages will be painful to the touch as you begin your treatment. This pain is a signal that you are already doing a good job dispersing the toxins and restoring the healing electromagnetic forces to their full power.

You can practise Zone Therapy on yourself, or sometimes it is more convenient to get other people to practise it on you. If you are practising it on yourself and you are supple enough, the seating position illustrated in the photograph opposite with your foot on your knee is the most natural:

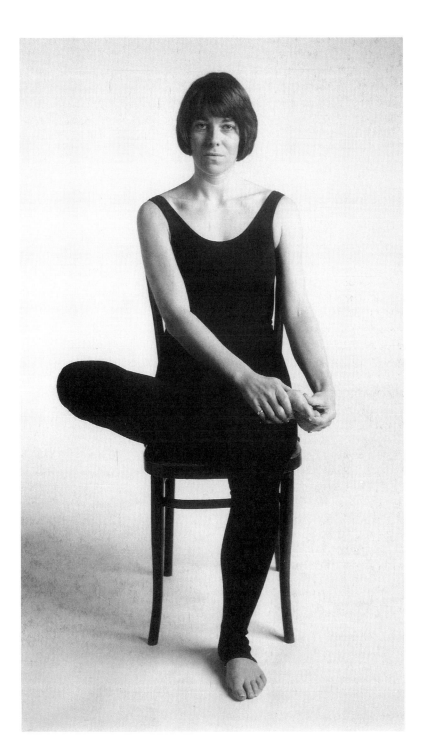

If this is uncomfortable
(perhaps your backache means
you are not supple enough)
you may, on the other hand,
place your foot on a stool like
this:

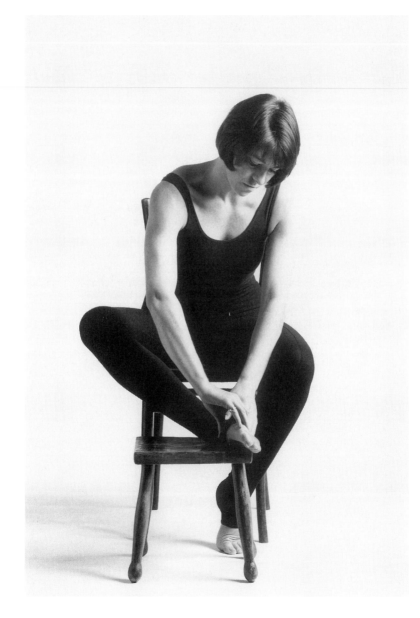

Some unfortunate people may be unable to reach their feet at all. In this case I recommend that you massage the pressure points on the underside of the foot by placing the foot on a golf ball on the floor and revolving the foot so that the ball rubs the pressure points. Obviously, in this case, though, ask someone else to perform the treatment on you if you can.

If someone else is treating you, the position illustrated below is the most natural one, and is the one I use in my clinic.

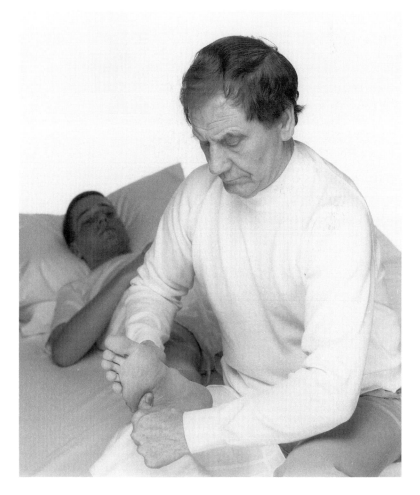

So use the top of the thumb, finger or rounded instrument, applying it to the point indicated in the diagrams that follow. Press into the point, rotating in a clockwise or anti-clockwise motion, whichever suits you. Always massage with an upward and outward circular movement. Do not let the thumb, finger or instrument slide over the surface of the skin. Rather, finish massaging one pressure point, then remove pressure altogether before moving on to the next one.

Massage the pressure points in the following sequence. Each rotation of the finger, thumb or instrument will take you approximately one second so that the number of seconds specified on each pressure point will also tell you the number of rotations required on each point. Then move to the next one. The complete massage will take approximately five minutes per foot. The positions of the pressure points are the same on each foot.

1) *Start by massaging the pressure points for the base of the spine which run along the ridge on the inside edge of the foot. Do this for twenty seconds. At each point massage down into the bone from above, on the bone and then up into the bone from below.*

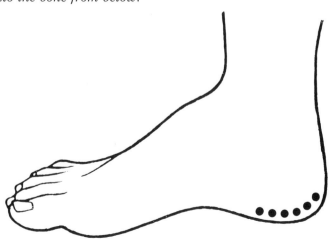

2) Continue massaging the ridge through the middle area of the foot which contains the pressure points for the lumbar area of the back. Do this for twenty seconds.

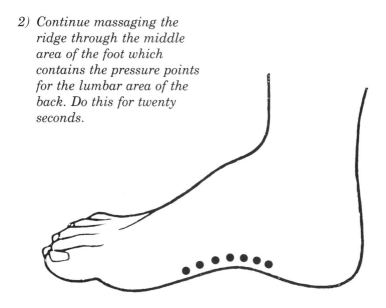

3) Massage the pressure points along the ridge as it goes over the ball of the foot – these cover the upper lumbars and the seventh cervical. Again for twenty seconds.

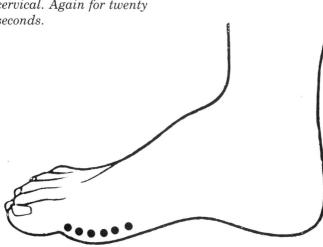

4) *Continue to massage the pressure points which lie along the ridge of the big toe, covering the cervicals and the back of the neck for twenty seconds.*

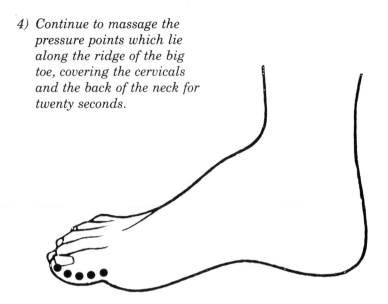

5) *Then work for ten seconds all over the top of the big toe from the joint to the base of the toenail; the skin across the big toe is thin so use your thumb or finger here rather than a rounded instrument. This part of the treatment brings relief to the back of the neck.*

6) *Work for twenty seconds across the top of the foot where the toes join the foot, working from the big toe towards the little toe, working also in the spaces between the toes. This will disperse toxins which cause tension and pain in the upper back of the neck and the shoulders.*

7) *Work again for twenty seconds across the foot but this time about one inch from where the toes join the feet. This treatment is for the upper and centre back and also for the shoulder and shoulder joints.*

8) Work again for twenty seconds across the foot but this time around the middle of the foot – this affects the middle of the back.

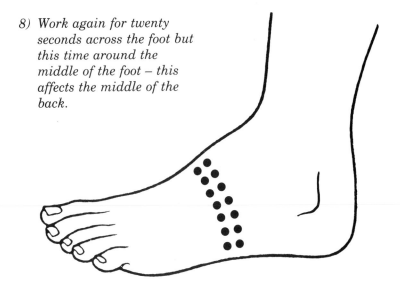

9) Work across the top of the foot near the join with the leg – this will give you wonderful freedom from pain and discomfort around the neck, shoulders and upper centre back. Twenty seconds.

10) Now work along the top of the foot from the base of the big toe down to the ankle – this is excellent for both the top and lower back. Twenty seconds.

11) Work along the other edge of the foot from the joint of the small toe to the ankle – this gives relief from the shoulder point through the rib cage down to the hips and lower back. Twenty seconds.

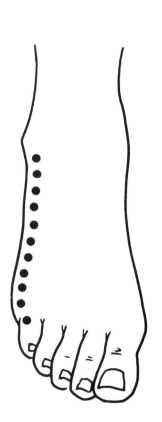

12) On the bottom of the foot now, work around the edge of the heel – again this is excellent for the lower back. Twenty seconds.

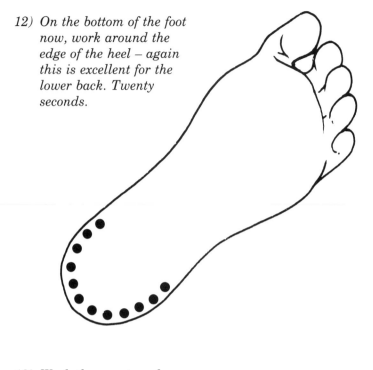

13) Work the very top of every toe – this helps the flow of healing power through all ten zones. Ten seconds.

14) *Work the nerve endings on the outer edge of the foot between the ridge of the heel and the ankle – these are very important for the back and hip. Ten seconds.*

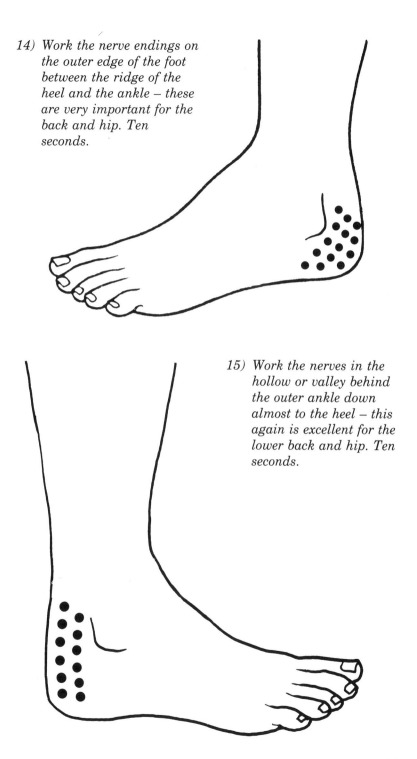

15) *Work the nerves in the hollow or valley behind the outer ankle down almost to the heel – this again is excellent for the lower back and hip. Ten seconds.*

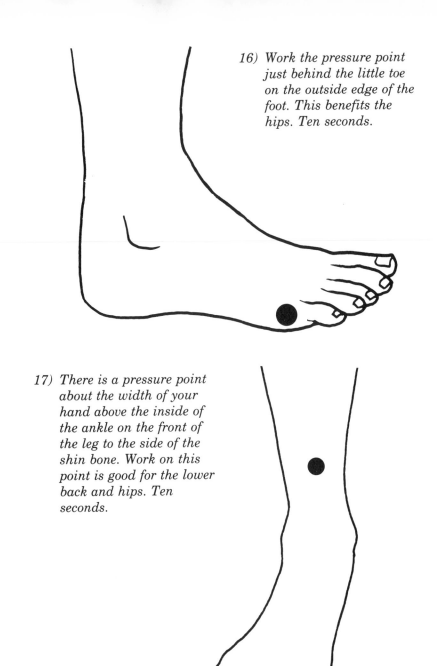

16) Work the pressure point just behind the little toe on the outside edge of the foot. This benefits the hips. Ten seconds.

17) There is a pressure point about the width of your hand above the inside of the ankle on the front of the leg to the side of the shin bone. Work on this point is good for the lower back and hips. Ten seconds.

18) *The nerve ending in the centre of the back of the knee is excellent for the lower back and lumbago, but do not massage this pressure point if you have varicose veins in this area. Ten seconds.*

19) *Work the pressure point which is approximately four fingers' width below the kneecap and one inch to the side of the bone on the outside of the leg. This benefits the back all the way down the side. Ten seconds.*

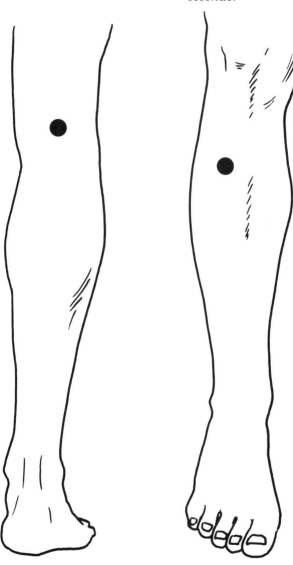

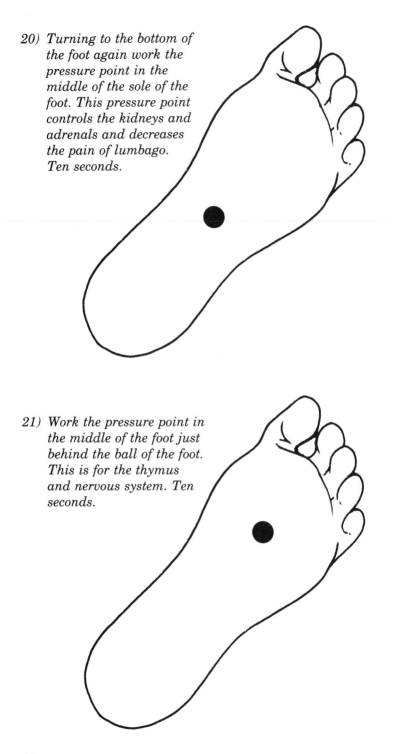

20) *Turning to the bottom of the foot again work the pressure point in the middle of the sole of the foot. This pressure point controls the kidneys and adrenals and decreases the pain of lumbago. Ten seconds.*

21) *Work the pressure point in the middle of the foot just behind the ball of the foot. This is for the thymus and nervous system. Ten seconds.*

22) Work for twenty seconds on the pressure points on the bottom of the foot where the toes join the foot. Work all the soreness out of these areas and you will feel great relief in the neck and shoulders and the top of the back.
Next work the same twenty-two pressure points on the other foot.

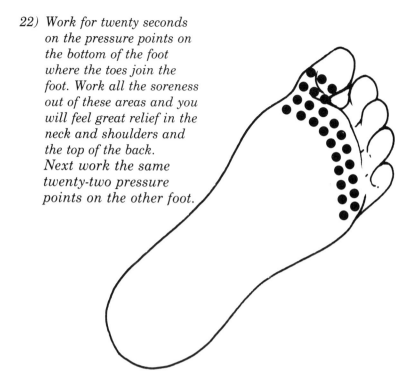

You have just completed a thorough work-out of your whole back, shoulders and neck. This part of the treatment should have taken approximately ten minutes. Now it is time to return to the area of particular pain, not only to work on the relevant pressure points for the particular vertebrae affected but also to work on the pressure points for the glands and organs closely connected with those vertebrae.

Zone Therapy for backache in specific areas

Pain in the First Cervical

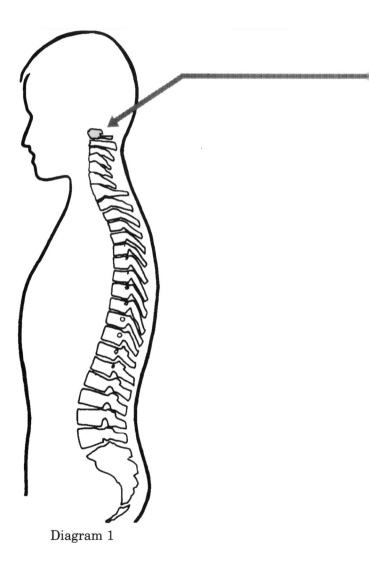

Diagram 1

If you are suffering from pain in the first cervical – see diagram 1 – you must work on and around the pressure points for the first cervical on the edge of the right foot – see diagram 2. Press as hard as you can bear and as precisely as you can on the pressure points and rotate your finger. If the pain becomes unbearable move your finger to points slightly above or below the pressure points for a few seconds, massage these areas, then move back to the pressure points. Keep this up for five minutes. Secondly, massage the pressure points on the soles of the feet for the glands and organs closely related to the first cervical as indicated on diagram 2; in this case they are the brain, the scalp, the ear, the eye, the nasal passages, the heart and the stomach. Repeat process on the left foot. Spend ten minutes on each foot.

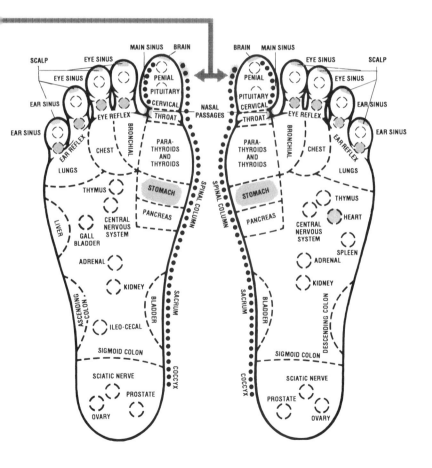

Diagram 2

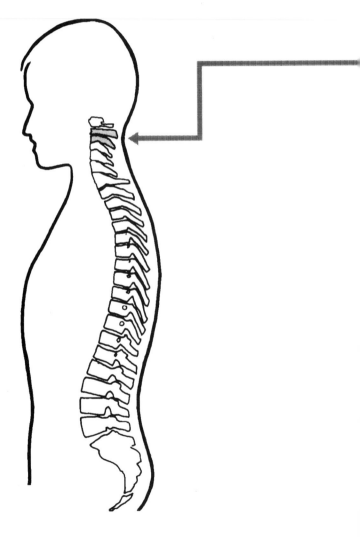

Work on the pressure points for the second and third cervicals on the right foot by using the method described on page 31. Then massage the pressure points on the sole of the foot for the connected glands and organs: the heart, the stomach, the diaphragm and the solar plexus. Again repeat process on the left foot spending ten minutes on each foot.

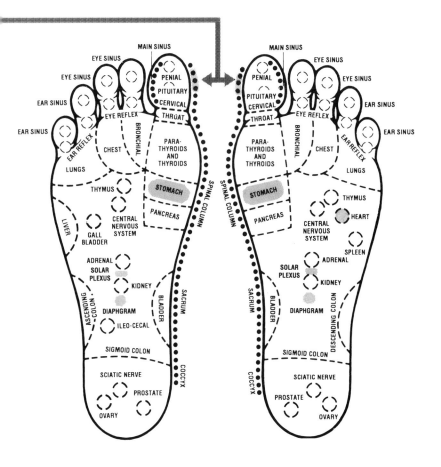

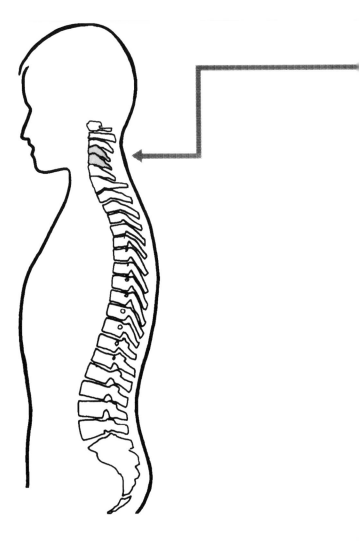

Do the following massage first on the right then on the left foot. Work for twenty minutes on the pressure points for the fourth and fifth cervicals and then on the pressure points for the connected glands and organs: the thyroid glands, the throat, the heart, the diaphragm, the liver and the stomach.

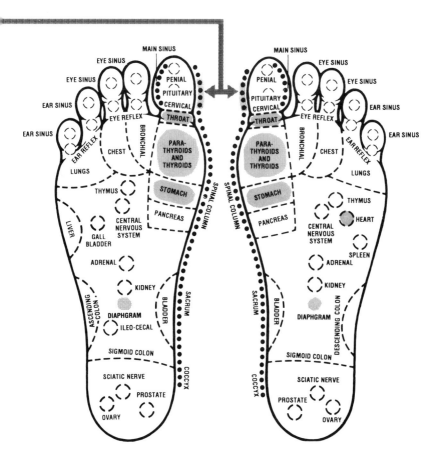

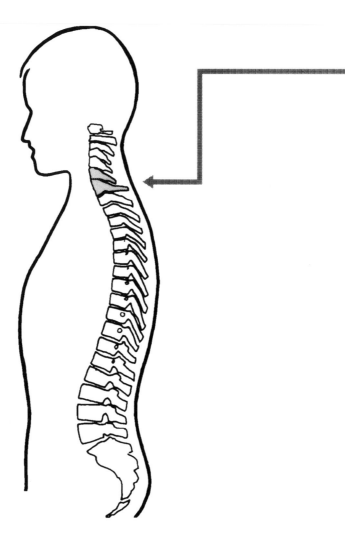

Do the following massage first on the right then on the left foot. Work for twenty minutes on the pressure points for the sixth and seventh cervicals and then on the pressure points for the connected glands and organs: the thyroid glands, the bronchial tubes, the throat, the chest and the heart.

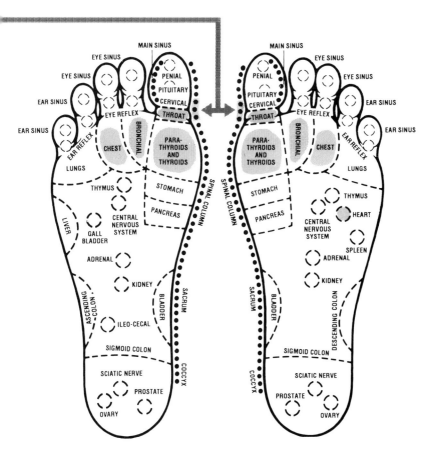

Pain in the First and Second Dorsals

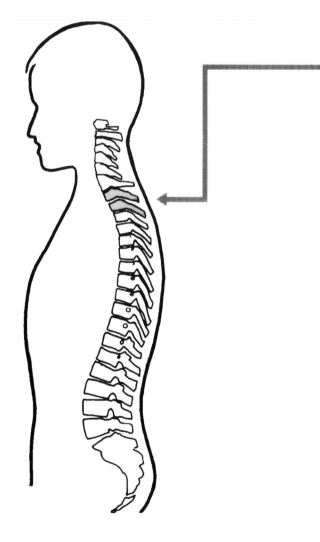

Do the following massage first on the right then on the left foot. Work for twenty minutes on the pressure points for the first and second dorsals and then on the pressure points for the connected glands and organs: the heart, the lungs, the bronchial tubes, the eyes and the ears.

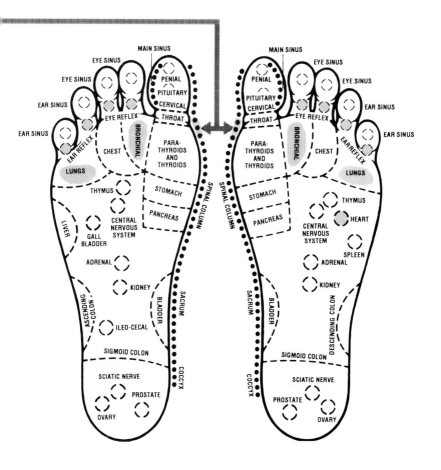

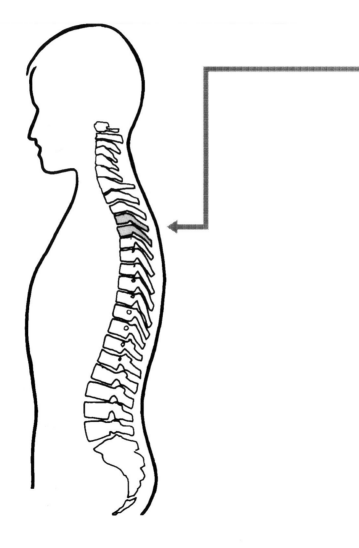

Do the following massage first on the right then on the left foot. Work for twenty minutes on the pressure points for the third and fourth dorsals and then on the pressure points for the connected glands and organs: the heart, the brain, the diaphragm, the stomach, the lungs, the ears, the eyes and the bronchial tubes.

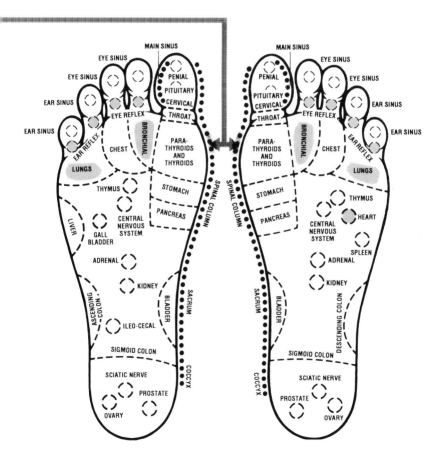

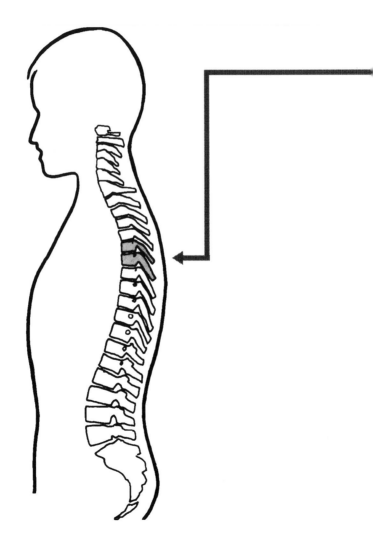

Do the following massage first on the right then on the left foot. Work for twenty minutes on the pressure points for the fifth and sixth dorsals and then on the pressure points for the connected glands and organs: the heart, the stomach, the lungs, the spleen, the ears, the eyes, the chest, the brain and the throat.

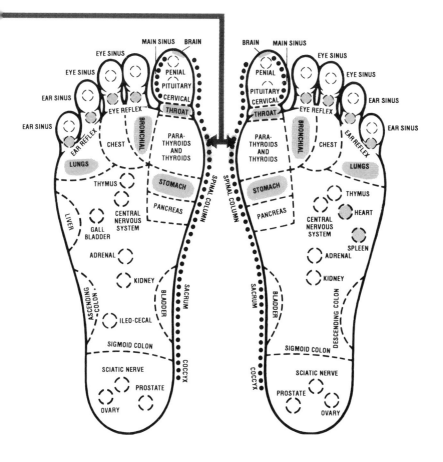

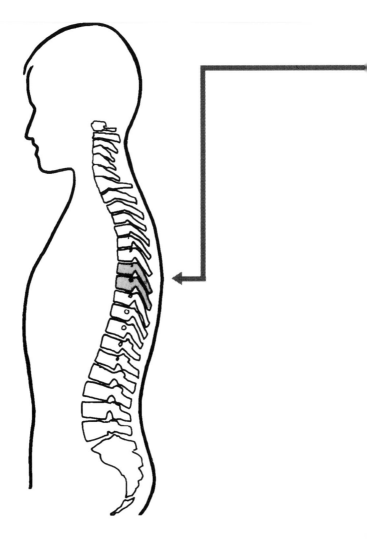

Do the following massage first on the right then on the left foot. Work for twenty minutes on the pressure points for the seventh and eighth dorsals and then on the pressure points for the connected glands and organs: the spleen, the pancreas, the intestines, the liver, the stomach and the kidneys.

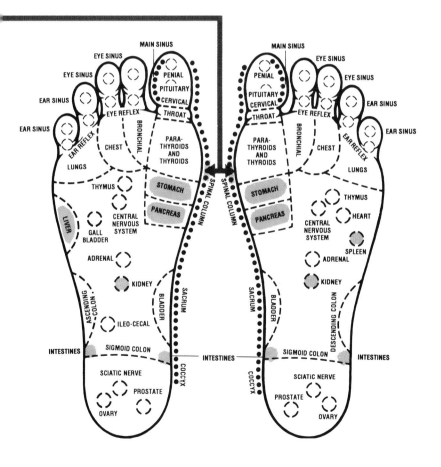

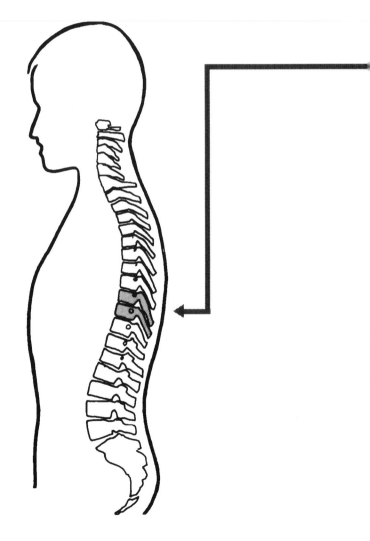

Do the following massage first on the right then on the left foot. Work for twenty minutes on the pressure points for the ninth and tenth dorsals and then on the pressure points for the connected glands and organs: the kidneys, the pancreas, the liver, and the adrenals.

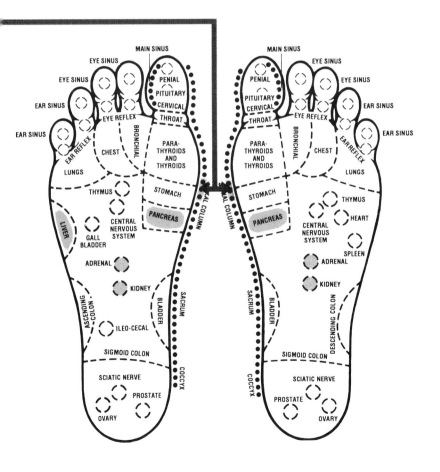

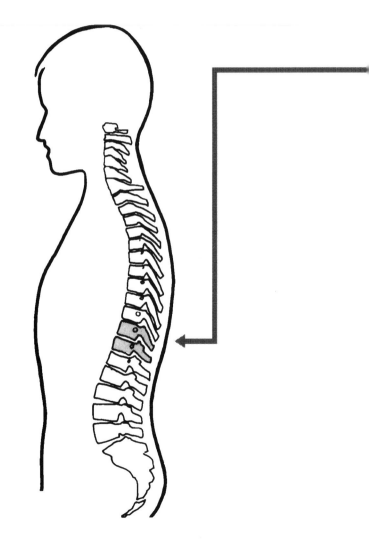

Do the following massage first on the right then on the left foot. Work for twenty minutes on the pressure points for the eleventh and twelfth dorsals and then on the pressure points for the connected glands and organs: the kidneys, the intestines, the bladder, the prostate gland, the throat, the rectum, the testes and the ovaries.

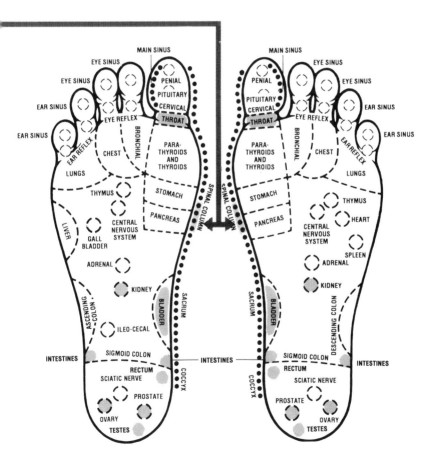

Lumbago: Pain in the First and Second Lumbars

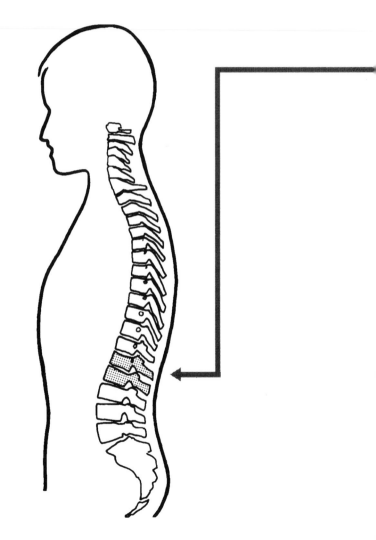

Do the following massage first on the right then on the left foot. Work for twenty minutes on the pressure points for the first and second lumbars and then on the pressure points for the connected glands and organs: the bladder, the kidneys, the intestines, the prostate gland, the sexual organs, the brain and the rectum.

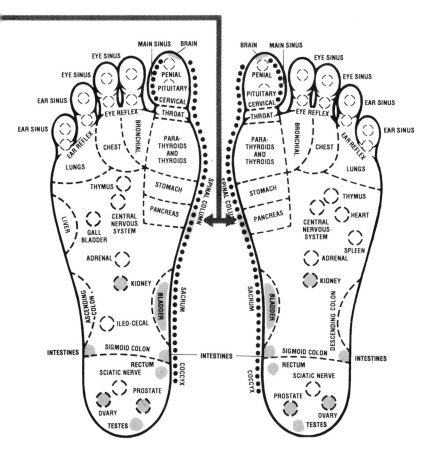

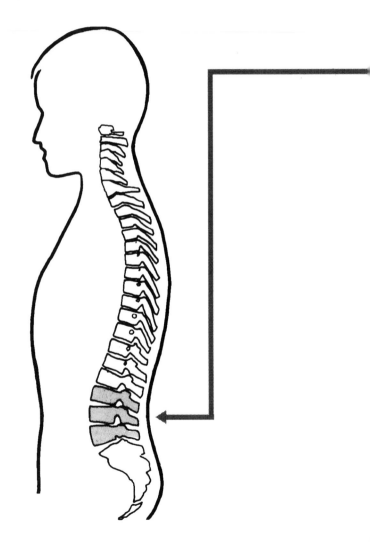

Do the following massage first on the right then on the left foot. Work for twenty minutes on the pressure points for the third, fourth and fifth lumbars and then on the pressure points for the connected glands and organs: the sexual organs, the ovaries, the intestines, the rectum, the prostate gland, and the bladder.

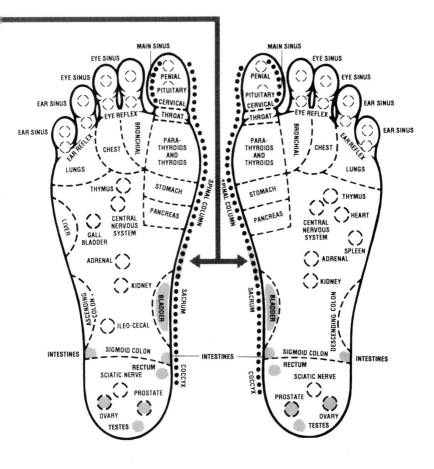

Supplementary exercises for the hands and the head

Working on the pressure points on the feet is the most direct way of using Zone Therapy to attack back pain. However, if your back pain is so bad that you cannot reach your feet and if no one else is available to perform the massage on you, you should, as well as doing as much as you can by rubbing the soles of your feet with a golf ball (see p. 17), work on the corresponding pressure points on your hands. Also, even if you are able to work regularly and fully on your feet it is a good idea to work on the pressure points on your hands at odd times during the day; for example, if you find yourself waiting for a train or a bus or sitting in a traffic queue. In addition there are a couple of exercises you can usefully perform on the head.

Again, massage the pressure points in the following sequence. Unless otherwise specified spend ten seconds, that's ten rotations of the finger, thumb or rounded instrument, on each point, then move to the next one. The complete massage will take 7½ minutes per hand. The pressure points are the same on each hand.

1) *Start massaging the pressure points for the base of the spine which run along the ridge on the inside edge of the hand where the hand joins the wrist.*

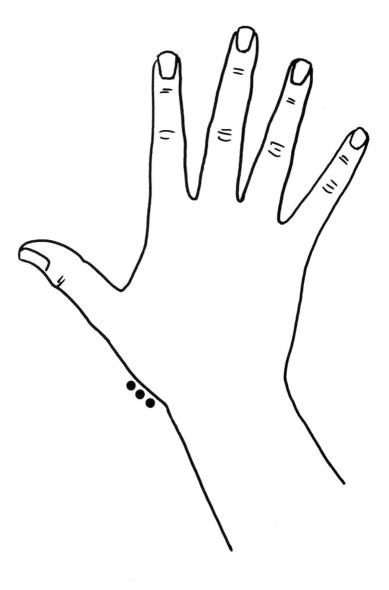

2) *Continue massaging the ridge running along the middle area of the hand which contains the pressure points for the lumbar area of the back – any congestion here will also affect the bladder and the kidneys.*

3) Massage the pressure
   points along the ridge as it
   goes over the palm of the
   hand – these cover the
   upper lumbars and the
   seventh cervical.

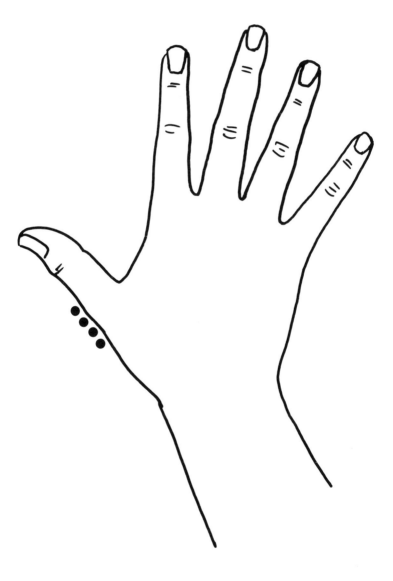

4) *Continue to massage the
pressure points which lie
along the ridge of the
thumb, covering the
cervicals and the back of
the neck.*

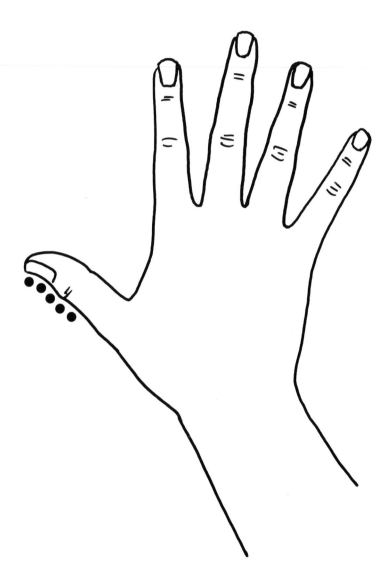

5) *Massage the ridge on the opposite side of the hand from the top of the little finger, down the side of the finger and the hand to the wrist. This is excellent for the rib cage, the shoulders, hips, sciatica and lumbago.*

6) Turning the hand over, work the valley between the thumb and the forefinger down as far as the bottom of the thumb where it joins the wrist.

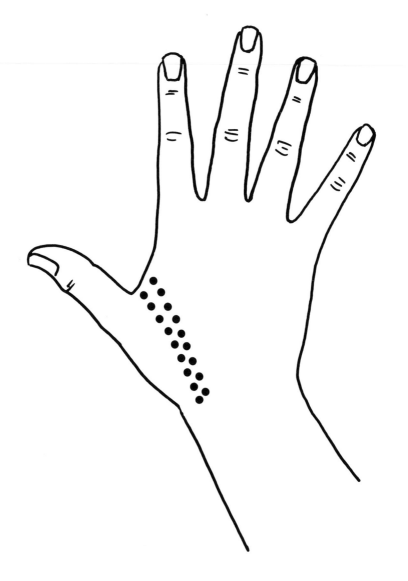

7) *Massage intensively the*
   valleys between the fingers
   as far down as the wrist.
   This does wonders for
   backache.

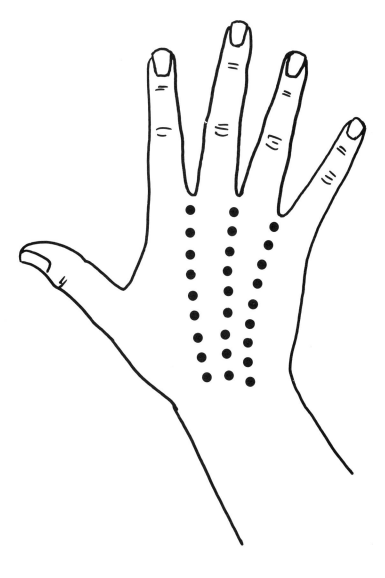

8) *Work all over the back of the hand, massaging all the way down to the wrist. This is good for any form of backache, particularly muscular backache.*

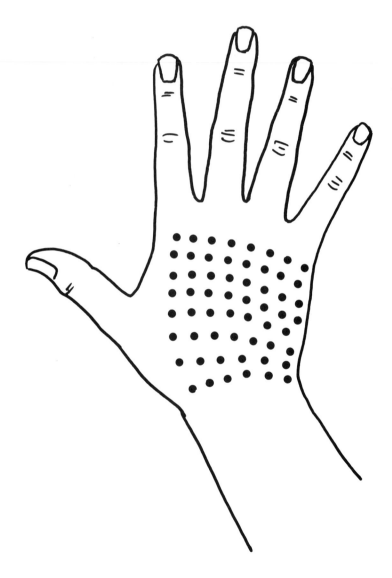

9) Work the nerve on the top of the hand midway between the knuckles and the wrist in the valley between the third and little fingers.

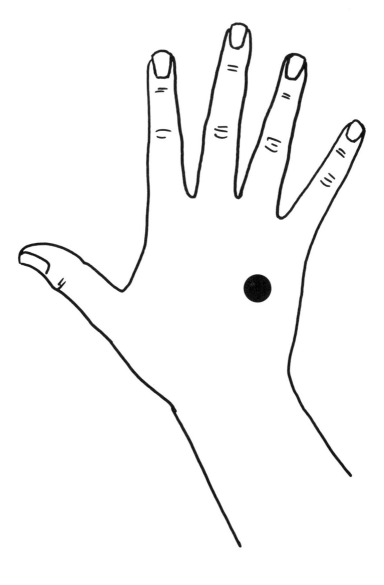

10) *Work the webbing between the thumb and forefinger. Then close the thumb to the forefinger and massage in the valley. This is excellent for the neck and shoulders.*

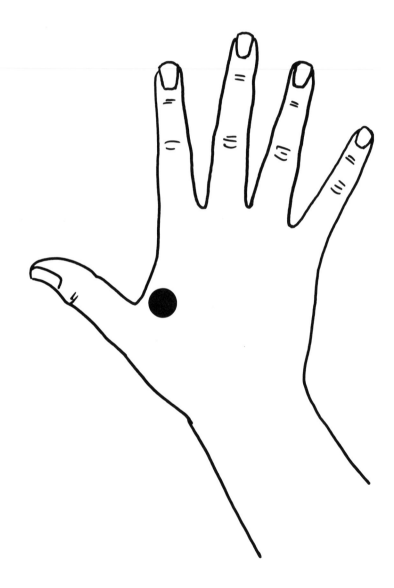

*11) Work down the outside
edge of the thumb on the
joint for the first, second
and third cervicals.*

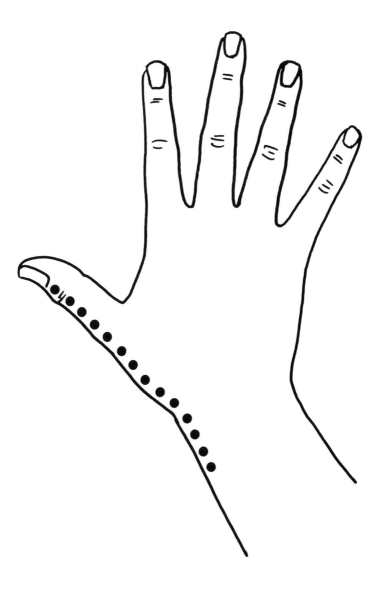

12) Press the teeth of a
common painted
aluminium comb all over
the palms of the hands
and the thumb areas. Do
this for five minutes to
achieve the best results.

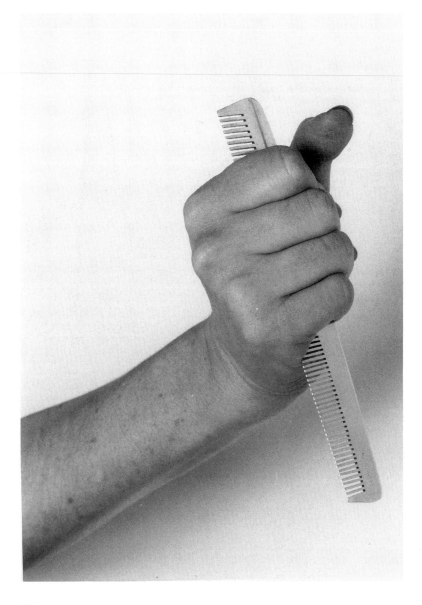

13) *Massage the pressure point below the eyebrow over the centre of the eye for the lower back and neck. Use little pressure.*

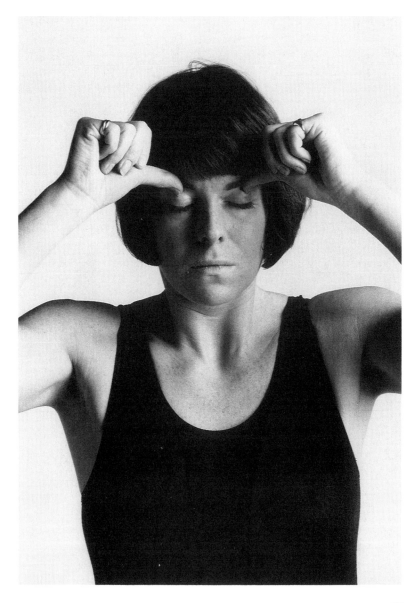

*14) Work the pressure point
on the spine on the upper
back between the first and
second dorsal vertebrae
parallel to the shoulders.
This is good for the neck
and shoulders.*

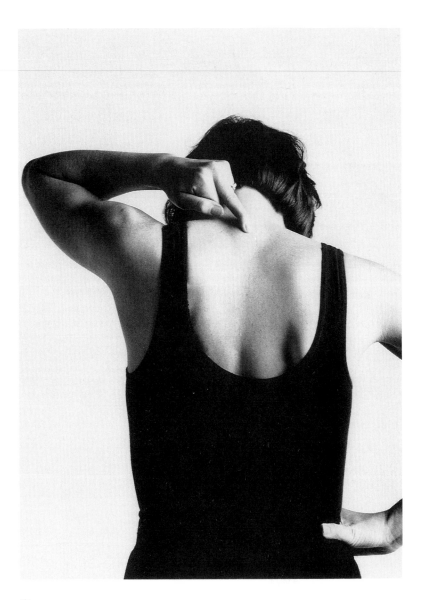

15) *The tongue is split into ten zones, five on either side of the middle of the tongue. So the middle of the tongue represents the spinal column. The front of the tongue is the head and neck and as you go further back you go down through the shoulders, middle of the back and on to the waist and lower back. Spend ten seconds working down the centre of your tongue.*

Special Problems

Osteoporosis

Osteoporosis is a condition where the density of the bone is diminished. It is usually found in women who have a low bone mass after the menopause. In fact this accounts for around 75 per cent of all cases. It is a major health problem. Indeed half as many women will die as a result of hip fracture as will die of breast cancer.

In literal terms 'osteo' means bone and 'porosis' originates from the Greek word *poros* meaning cavity formation. When viewed under magnification, normal bone will be seen to be similar to a honeycomb structure with hollow inner cavities. It is this formation which gives it its great strength in much the same way that metal tubes strategically placed will take enormous loads. However, if rust is allowed to erode the metal then inevitably its strength diminishes to the point where it will break up; the softening of cavity structures which takes place during osteoporosis will have a similar effect.

Although osteoporosis has reached epidemic proportions there are ways of beating it. In the first instance women should ensure that they have a diet that is rich in calcium before and during pregnancy and especially while breast-feeding, when the body loses four times its normal calcium loss during lactation.

Women who are entering or who have passed through the menopausal stage of life are at the most risk from calcium insufficiency, particularly if calcium has not been a significant ingredient of their diet since childhood and if they have breast-fed children without extra calcium intake during the pregnancy and lactating period.

In fact, there are many people who need a calcium supplement to provide an optimum level to avoid serious health problems. Intake is not the end of this matter. Absorption makes all the difference between being calcium sufficient and showing signs of an insufficiency. If calcium is not absorbed through the walls of the small intestine into the bloodstream and then circulated through the bodily systems to replace that lost from the bones then, obviously, it is of little value.

So, it is essential when seeking a good calcium supplement to choose one in which the calcium is easily absorbed. There is little doubt among nutritionists that calcium citrate is absorbed better than any other form of calcium. So check your supplement label to ensure that calcium citrate is the first item on the ingredient list. Do not be confused by an overall large quantity of calcium on a nutritional information panel. Remember it is the amount absorbed which is vital and not the intake.

No calcium supplement is worth its salt when dealing with bone porosis or building and strengthening bones unless it contains Vitamin D. Vitamin D is essential for growing and maintaining healthy bones and teeth since it greatly helps the absorption of calcium. Select a calcium citrate with half as much magnesium citrate, some Boron and Vitamin D for the best results.

Back Pain and Arthritis
Arthritis is a factor which affects quite a percentage of back problems.

One of the most encouraging developments in recent years has been the discovery of a natural nutrient which has proved highly beneficial in the treatment of arthritis in back pain, joint pains, whip-lash and neuralgia.

It is the extract of the green-lipped mussel eaten daily by New Zealand Maoris. This species of mussel is rich in protein, minerals and other nutrients and one particular variety, *Perna Canaliculus*, is proving its value as a new natural remedy for back pain and arthritis.

Perna mussels have evolved a particularly efficient filter-feeding system that has been described as a marvel of nature. Sieving up to ten gallons of sea water daily, their bodies have become enriched with a unique blend of chelated minerals, vitamins, trace elements, amino acids and other nutrients.

Among them lies the secret of the green-lipped mussel extract's beneficial effect on joint inflammation. This seems to be a large protein molecule which attacks the root cause of arthritis and back pain as well as relieving the symptoms. The only problem that has arisen is the increase in pain that affects some people while the active nutrient is getting to work during the first weeks of treatment.

I have now overcome this problem with the development of pernamer. This formulation adds 75 mg of the pain-relieving amino acid DLPA (Phenylalanine) to the 350 mg of pure mussel extract in each capsule. The recommended daily dosage of pernamer is three capsules taken with food. Pernamer is non-addictive and its affects are cumulative. **Warning: you cannot take this pernamer extract if you are allergic to sea foods.**

If your poor old dog or cat suffers with arthritis in the back legs then try giving your pet the pernamer capsules and watch the magic transformation. You will have a young dog or cat again.

The pernamer formula is available in all good health stores throughout the UK.

Sciatica
The sciatic nerve comes out of the pelvis, runs along the back of the thigh and eventually divides into two. When this nerve becomes injured or inflamed, it can be extremely painful.

The sciatic pressure point on the foot is situated slightly to the outside of the centre of the heel, so if you start treatment to the feet in the centre of the heel and work along that line to the outside of the foot, you will find the tender area. You may need something a little more penetrating than your thumb or finger, and I would suggest the end of a rounded pencil. You will find another pressure point on the inside of the ankle and this should also receive attention. The sciatic pressure point on the hands is where the hand meets the wrist. Work all the way across this area, using only your finger and thumb. In addition, on both the hands and feet, massage all areas of the spinal column, particularly the lower lumbar, sacrum and coccyx, and also the colons and prostate or ovary. Whilst you are doing the treatment for five minutes a day on each hand and foot massaging each point for only ten seconds at a time, check out all the glands and organs to make sure all is well.

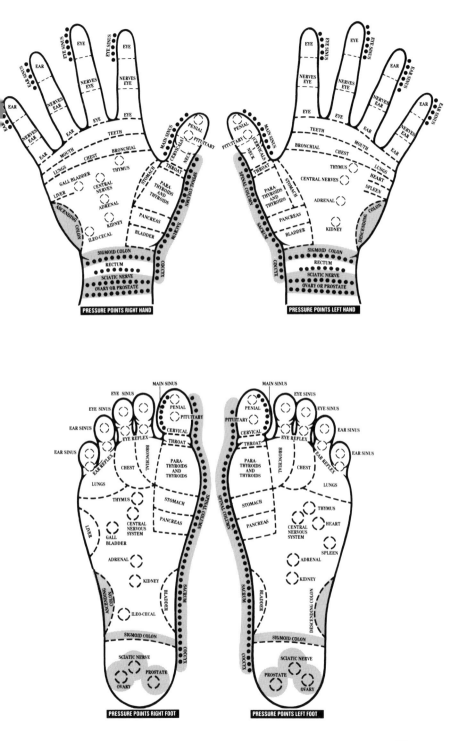

73

Exercises to strengthen the back

When you have cured your backache using Zone Therapy, you should persist with Zone Therapy in order to keep yourself in 100 per cent health and fitness.

You should also do some of the following exercises designed to strengthen your back. You want strong, firm muscles which give a wonderful contour to the body and enable you to perform most movements with ease and comfort. This is achieved through simple exercises. I must emphasize that *none of these exercises should be attempted until your back is completely cured* – if you are not sure, do not try them. In fact, you must check and consult your medical doctor before performing exercises. Especially if you have not had a recent medical check up, or if you smoke or drink, or if you are overweight, or you have specific medical problems, or there is heart disease in the family. Check with your doctor first. Even if your doctor gives you the all clear to begin with work at it gently and slowly, mastering one exercise at a time, until you are strong enough to do the harder exercises.

Your physical strength is determined by the strength of your muscles.

If you can manage to spend half an hour per day on these back-strengthening exercises *in addition to the practice of Zone Therapy*, you will go a long way towards avoiding future problems.

Exercise One

Stand with arms outstretched at shoulder level, your hands making loose fists. Rotate your shoulders back and down away from your ears. Do not let your shoulders or your arms drop. Do this for one full minute keeping your arms up and work well.

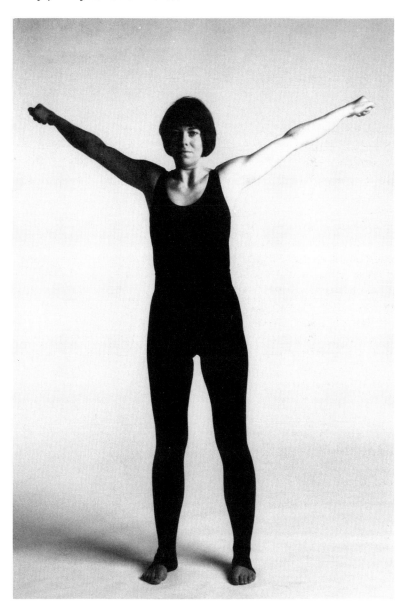

Exercise Two

*Stand against the wall,
keeping your back tight
against the wall. Bend your
knees and tilt your pelvis
upwards. Hold. Release.
Perform six times.*

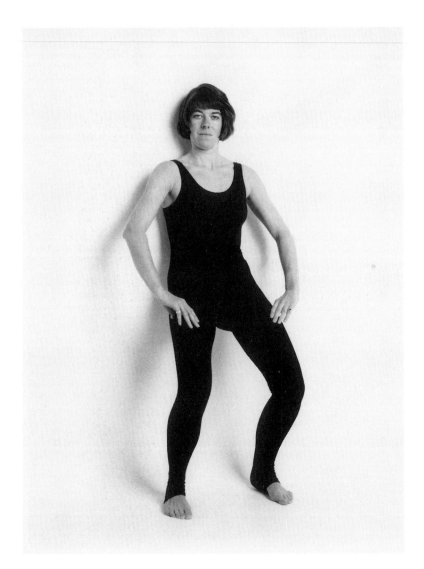

Exercise Three

Stand with your back to the wall, the heel of the left foot as near to the wall as possible. Place the right foot slightly in front of the left foot and stretch with your hands above the head, trying to touch the ceiling. Really stretch, stretch, stretch. Relax and repeat six times if you can do so without discomfort. Put some effort into it.

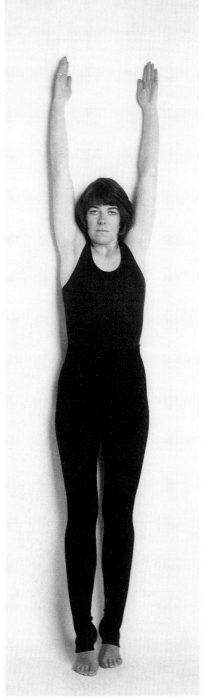

Exercise Four

Stand against the wall with your back flat against the wall and slowly try to go into a sitting position. Only go as far as you feel comfortable. Eventually you will really sit in the full position. Repeat three times.

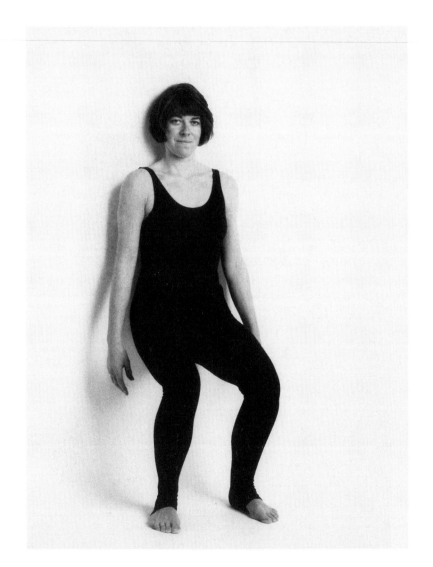

Exercise Five

If you have a table or desk against the wall, place the hands on the table and then stretch the legs far back. This is a modified version of floor press-ups which is easy to perform and very good. Get your hands and shoulders wide apart and your back as straight as possible. Do not arch your back. Bend both arms, bringing your chest to the table, then push up and straighten. Do six times or as many as possible without any strain.

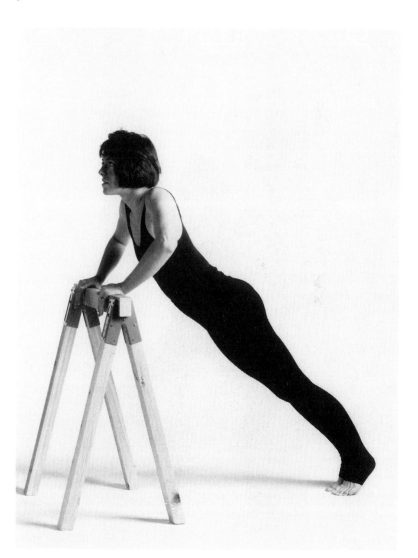

Exercise Six

Stand upright near a wall for support with your feet apart. Keep your back straight and your behind well tucked in. Stretch your arms out to the side of your body, feet pointed outwards, and do a deep knee bend. Keep your heels on the floor and return to starting position. Do this exercise six times. Do not, however, do this exercise if you have a bad knee problem.

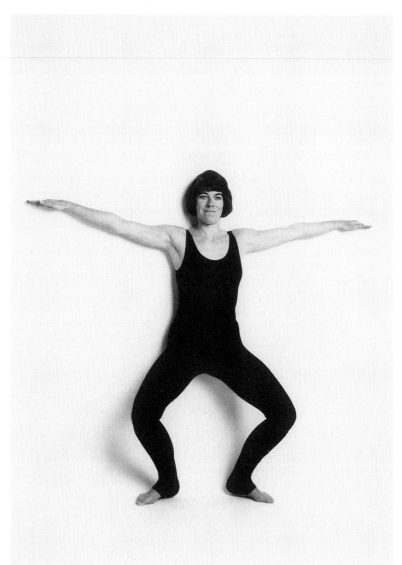

Exercise Seven

Sit on a chair or stool, back perfectly straight, feet firmly on the ground and weight evenly distributed. Now stretch your arms upwards as far as you can. Touch the ceiling in your mind. Relax for a moment, then stretch again. Do this exercise at least six times. You will feel the goodness of it.

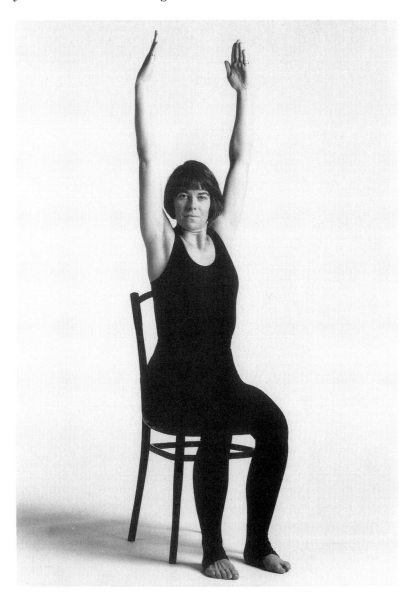

Exercise Eight

Sit on the chair obeying all the rules in the previous exercises. Now place your hands behind your head, fingers just touching. Lift your rib cage and mentally create as much space as you can between your neck and your hips, but do not mentally lift your shoulders.

Let your head drop on to your chest. Now, with the feeling of space between your neck and hips, force your head back with your hands resisting the pressure. It gives you a terrific feeling. Do six times.

The neck supports the weight of the head, and it is

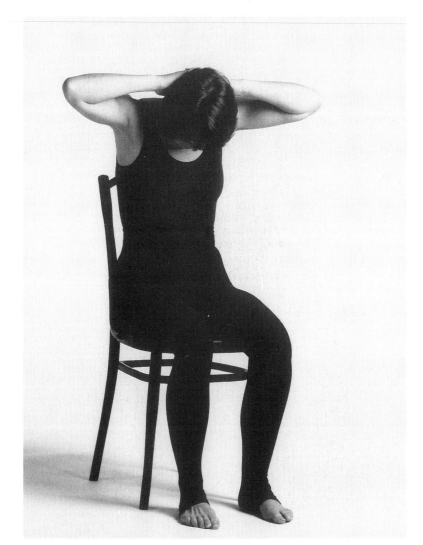

Exercise Nine

also a pathway for the blood vessels, the nervous system, respiratory and digestive systems. Tension in the neck is caused by anxiety, worry, stress and this can have serious implications for your general well being.

You can also give yourself a neck massage. Start by placing your hands on your shoulders as near to the neck as possible. Keep your fingers together and stroke firmly upwards.

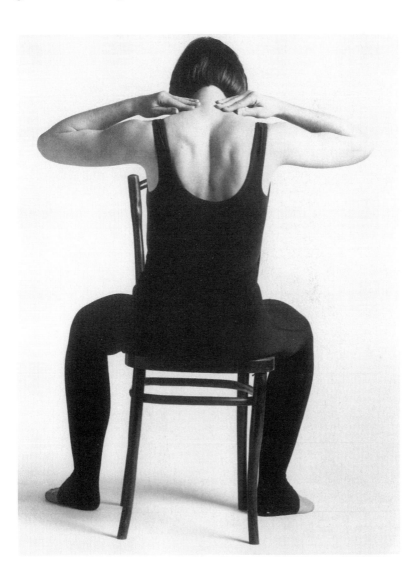

Exercise Ten

Massage deep into the base of
the neck and work out all the
tension, especially where the
head sits on the neck.

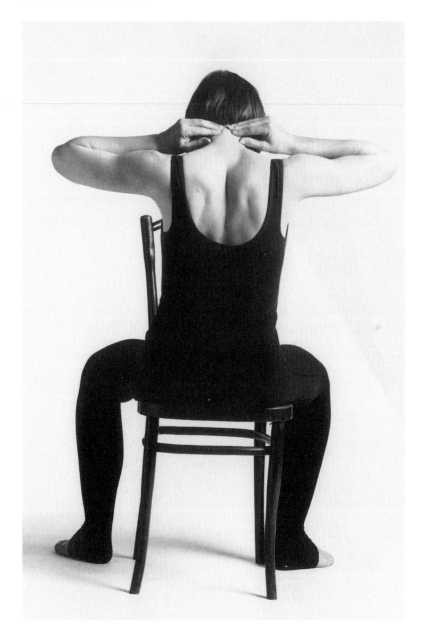

Exercise Eleven

Place one hand over the other
and massage into the neck
with the heel of both hands.

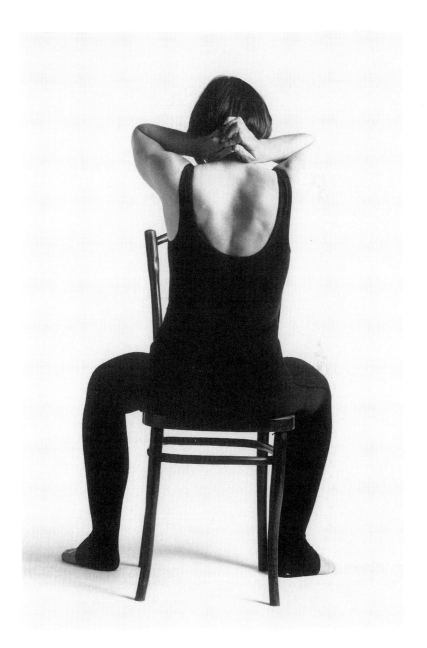

Exercise Twelve

Sitting down on a chair, rest both elbows on the side of the lower ribs. Keeping the elbows in position, pull back with the shoulders, arms and elbows.

This is a powerful exercise. Put some power into it and the results are great. Pull back strongly, several times.

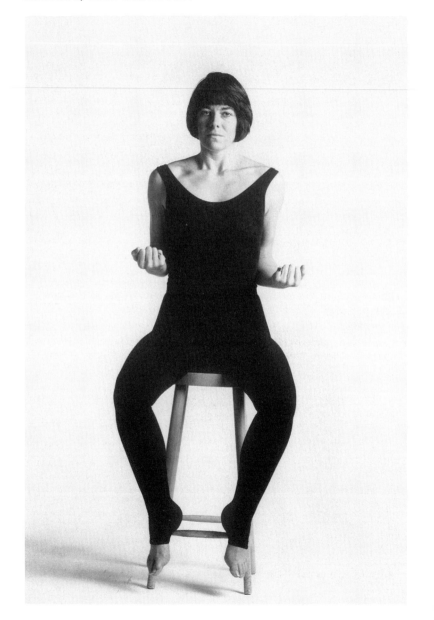

Exercise Thirteen

Sit on a chair, back as straight as possible, feet firmly on the ground. Place hands near the behind. Clasp hands together and pull the shoulder blades tightly together. Repeat twelve times.

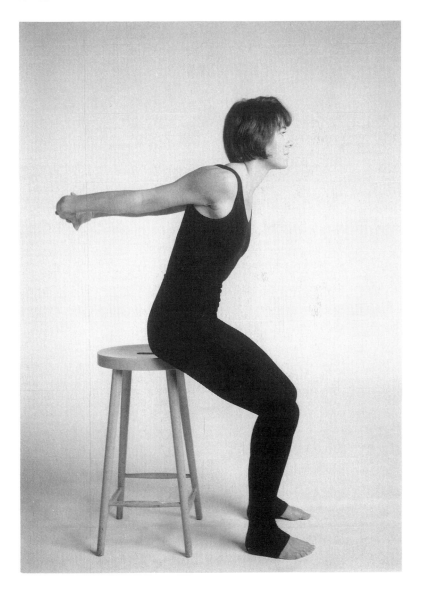

Exercise Fourteen

Sit on a chair, weight evenly distributed, feet firmly on the ground and the back perfectly straight. Stretch the arms out to the sides of the body at shoulder level. Make a fist and pull the shoulder blades together. Hold, then relax. Repeat twelve times if possible.

Exercise Fifteen

To exercise muscles around the waist, sit on a stool or chair, hands interlocked at the back of your head. Then bend over as far as possible to the right. Hold for five seconds and come back up into a straight position. Bend over to the left as far as possible. Hold for five

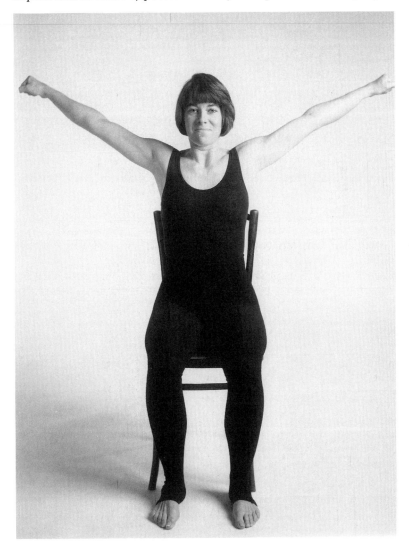

seconds and come back up into a straight position. Work this exercise so that you perform six bends to the right and six bends to the left. This will go a long way to making the muscles around the waist very strong and firm.

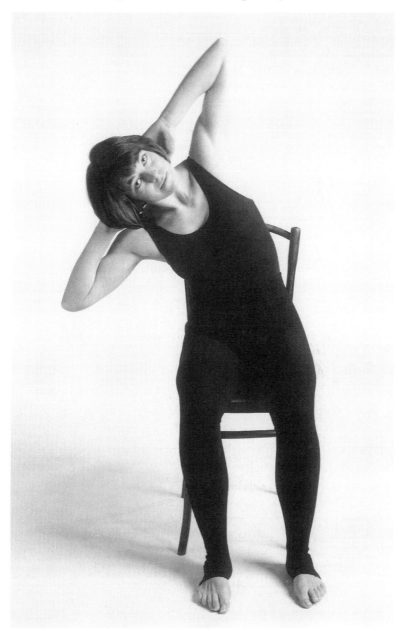

Exercise Sixteen

To exercise the stomach and the back, lie on the floor on your back with your hands on your thighs. Stretch your legs and feet and slide your hands down towards your knees at the same time. Bring up your head to look at your toes. Hold for five seconds and release. Repeat this exercise at least six times if you can do so without discomfort.

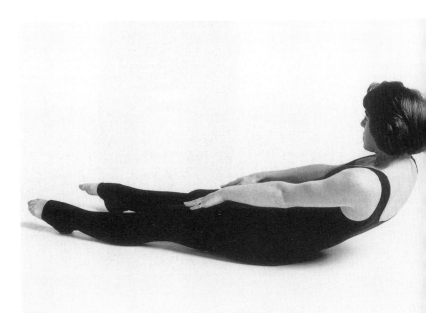

Exercise Seventeen

Now sit up with legs bent and feet and hips wide apart. Bring your chin towards your chest. Breathe out and lower your body backwards, pulling forwards with your arms and elbows at the same time. Hold it at the point where you feel your abdominal muscles going tight to prevent you from falling backwards. Repeat this exercise six times if you can without discomfort. It is terrific for the back and abdominal muscles.

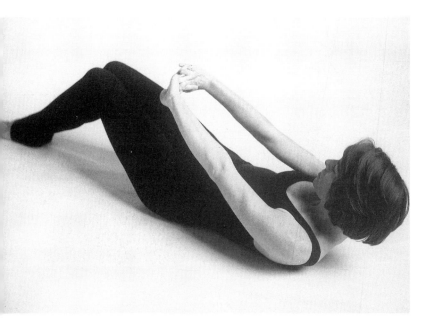

Exercise Eighteen

To strengthen the lower back, lie down, face downwards, with your forehead resting on your hands. Have your legs and hips wide apart. Then bend your legs and lift the right leg up. Hold it then return it to starting position and lift your leg up. Repeat on each leg six times if you can.

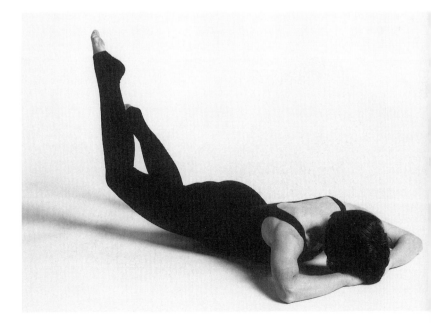

Exercise Nineteen

Still on the floor on your stomach, with your head resting on your hands, now straighten the legs. Lift the right leg straight six times, then the left leg straight six times.

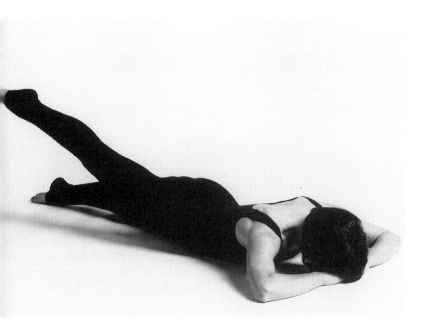

Exercise Twenty

Place a cushion under your pelvis to take the strain off the lower back. Then lift the right leg up. Hold for a few seconds then return to normal position and lift the left leg up and hold for a few seconds and return to normal. Practise this exercise at least six times on each leg.

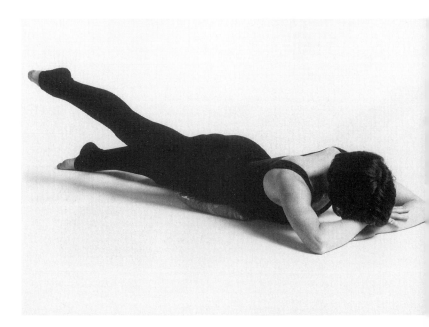

Exercise Twenty-one

Still in the same position with the cushion under your pelvis, now lift both legs as high as you comfortably can and hold the position for a few seconds, then return to normal. Do this exercise six times if possible.

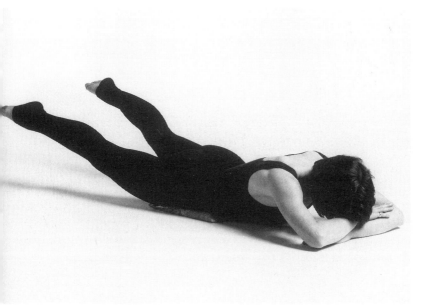

Exercise Twenty-two

*Take the cushion away, still
face down on the floor. Put
your hands behind you and
lift your head and chest off the
floor, keeping your feet on the
floor. Breathe in as you lift
your head and breathe out as
you lower your head. Repeat
six times if possible.*

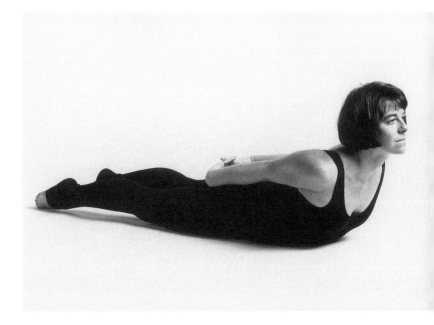

Exercise Twenty-three

*Still on the floor face down,
both legs straight, lift right
arm and left leg. Hold for five
seconds and relax. Lift left
arm and right leg and hold for
five seconds. Repeat six times
if possible.*

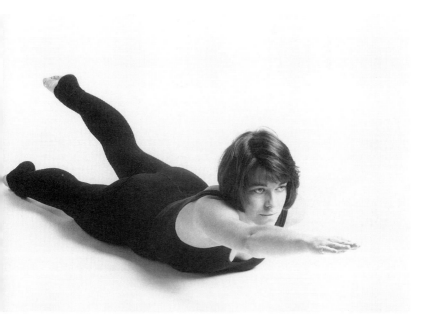

Exercise Twenty-four

Still on the floor face down, arms stretched out in front of you, legs in a straight line. Lift your hands and head off the floor as high as you can and at the same time lift your legs off the floor in a straight line and pull the legs up as high as you can. This is a powerful exercise for the back and you may also find that you can only manage maybe one or two in the beginning, but as you become stronger you will be able to do more.

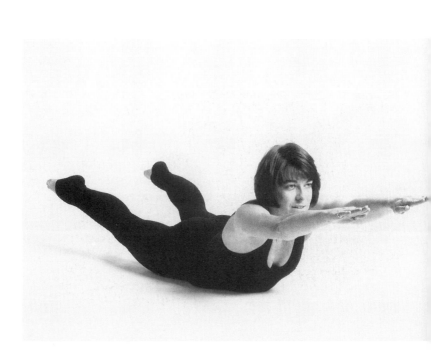

Exercise Twenty-five

Still on the floor face downwards, sit up on to the knees, then curl up into a ball with your head touching the floor and your face touching your knees, your arms stretching loosely behind you with wrists and hands near the feet and ankles. This is wonderfully relaxing.

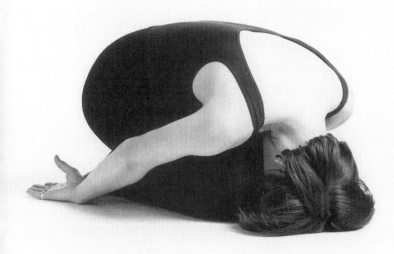

Exercise Twenty-six

Sit on the floor with your back straight, arms extended out to the sides of the body. Breathe in and bend forwards towards the feet. Attempt to keep the legs straight if possible and breathe out. The bend should come directly from the hips. Breathe in and return to starting point. Repeat six times if you can.

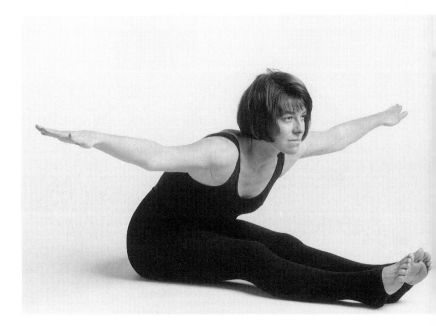

Exercise Twenty-seven

*Lie on the floor, knees in a
semi-bend, fingers interlocked,
palms facing outwards. Pull
with your hands and arms,
lifting your head and chest off
the floor and attempting to
bring your head and chest to
your knees. Repeat six times if
possible.*

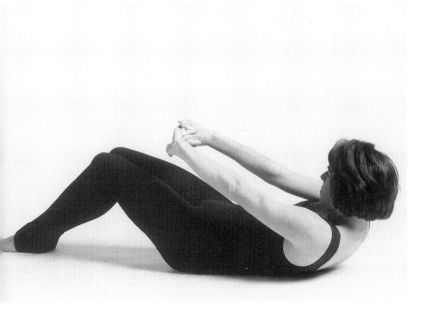

Exercise Twenty-eight

With both knees on the floor and hands on the floor, breathe in and lift the right leg as high as possible. Breathe out and return to normal position whilst lowering the leg. Look upwards. Then do the same exercise with the left leg. Repeat six times if possible.

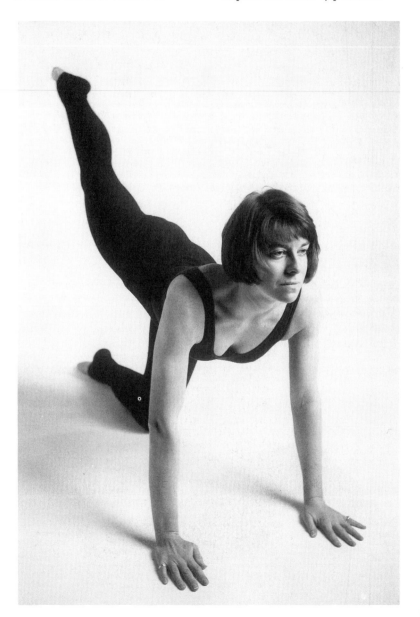

Exercise Twenty-nine

Still in the same position, knees on the floor and hands on the floor with arms straight, lift left leg as high as possible at the same time lowering the elbows and chin to the floor. Come back to normal position and do the same exercise lifting the right leg. Repeat six times if you can.

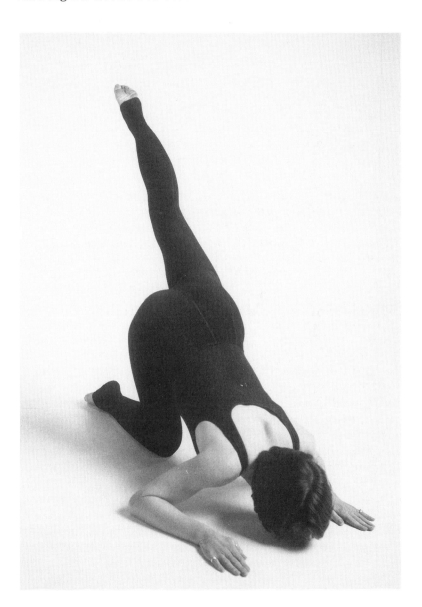

Improve your posture

After you have used Zone Therapy to cure yourself of the pain, correct posture is vital for helping you keep free of back problems.

Your head weighs about twelve pounds and how you hold it influences the position of the vertebrae all the way down the spine. So, to hold your head correctly, you have to imagine a spring attached to the top of your head which is taut and pulling upwards all the time so that the back of your neck lengthens.

Do not hold your neck in a rigid fashion; everything must be relaxed but straight as if you are being pulled up to the sky. Remember that strained neck muscles lead to headaches and other problems, so get the feeling of being like a puppet on a string.

At the same time you must relax your shoulders, let them drop, keep your eyes facing straight ahead and relax the muscles in your face completely.

Aches and pains in the upper back are mostly caused by holding the shoulders incorrectly. Most people sit or stand with one shoulder higher than the other. Bring them level by standing with your weight evenly balanced on both feet and holding your head upright. Look at your arms as an extension of the shoulders, letting them hang in a loose, relaxed manner by your side. Wrists and fingers should also be loose. Mentally create as much space as you can between your ribs and hips; keep your shoulders down and your back lengthened; this will help your digestive system to work better and your breathing will improve enormously. Work on the feeling that there is a great deal of space between the base of your head down to your coccyx.

When sitting down, on a chair, keep the spine lengthened and extended. Sit well back on it with your weight evenly distributed on both your buttocks, with both feet on the floor and your back in a straight line. Keep your thighs parallel.

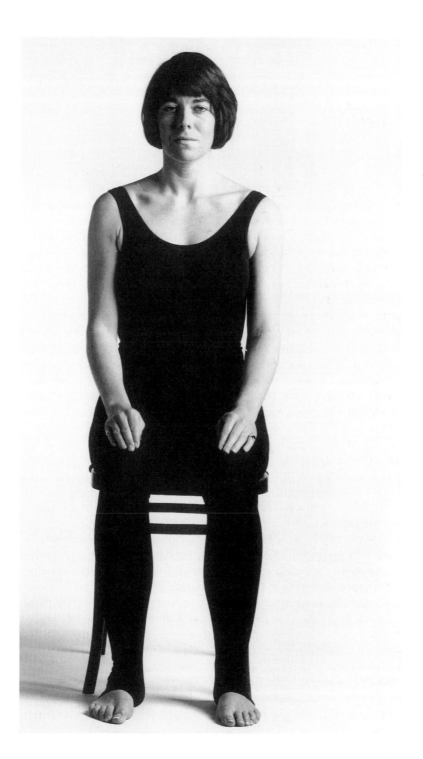

When you are sitting down, you may not be as comfortable as you may think. In fact the strain on your back may be dramatic. There is twice as much strain on your back when sitting as compared to standing. Prolonged sitting weakens the muscles and ligaments that support the spine, so if you are at a desk for hours at a time, do not lean towards your work, keep as upright as possible. Bring the work towards you. When you bend, whatever you are doing, make sure the bend either comes from the knees or from a natural swing of the hips. The spine must be kept straight just the same as it is when you are upright.

Bending from the lower back is one of the biggest contributors to major backache and severely strained back muscles. Remember this when you are making bends. Bend your knees to lift heavy things including children, and when gardening.

When you feel like relaxing do not flop into a chair. Lie flat on your back with your head resting on a couple of telephone directories. This will extend your spine and also will take all the strain out of your back. This is the best way to rest and relax your body. While lying down, bend your knees from time to time.

When you hold yourself correctly, your pelvis supports your spine and takes the pressure off your lower back. When walking or running or even standing your knees must not be rigid, they should be a little bit flexed to take the weight off your body and act as shock absorbers. This will help to prevent jarring. The following exercise is for posture.

Tree Exercise

Take up the tree position. Stand up in a straight line, feet together, hands stretched full length above your head, palms inwards, fingers relaxed, eyes open. Place the left foot as high as possible and as far as possible on to the right leg inner thigh. You should feel comfortable enough to stay there for at least one full minute.

Now close your eyes. If you feel yourself beginning to topple or fall over you know that your sense of balance needs attention, so you should practise this exercise until you stay perfectly balanced. Try this exercise up against the wall to begin with. After working the left foot on the right thigh, you must then practise the right foot up on the left thigh. Work away until you succeed.

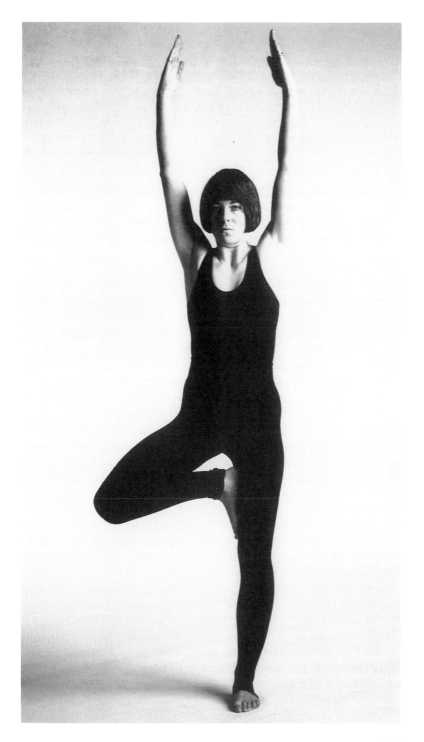

Breathing Properly

Life is absolutely dependent upon the act of breathing. Breath is life. To breathe is to live. Without breath there is no life.

The extraordinary thing is that very few men or women do breathe properly. Intelligent control of your breathing power will lengthen your days upon this earth by giving you increased vitality and powers of resistance.

Modern man has concocted improper methods and attitudes of walking, standing and sitting, which have robbed him of his birthright of natural and correct breathing. The results are shown in contracted chests and stooping shoulders and the terrible diseases of the respiratory organs.

It is estimated that in twenty-four hours, 35,000 pints of blood traverse the capillaries of the lungs, the blood corpuscles being exposed to the oxygen of the air on both of their surfaces. Unless fresh air in sufficient quantities reaches the lungs, the stream of blood cannot be purified, and consequently not only is the body robbed of its nourishment, but the waste products which should have been destroyed are returned to the circulation and poison the system. Death ensues or a state of imperfect health is experienced. In imperfect or shallow breathing, only a portion of the lung cells are brought into play and a great portion of the lung capacity is lost, the system suffering in proportion to the amount of under-oxygenation. The blood of someone who breathes improperly is of a bluish dark colour, lacking the red richness of pure arterial blood; this often shows itself in a poor complexion. Proper breathing and a consequent good circulation, on the other hand, result in a clear, bright complexion.

The lower animals in their nature state breathe naturally and primitive man undoubtedly did the same. The abnormal manner of living adopted by civilized man – the shadow that follows upon civilization – has robbed us of our natural habit of breathing and the race has greatly suffered. To rectify bad breathing habits, do the following exercises daily:

Breathing Exercise 1

Stand erect. Place the hands on each side of the body as high up under the armpits as you can, thumbs reaching towards the back. Inhale a complete breath. Retain the air for a short while then gently squeeze the sides, slowly exhaling at the same time. Do this five times.

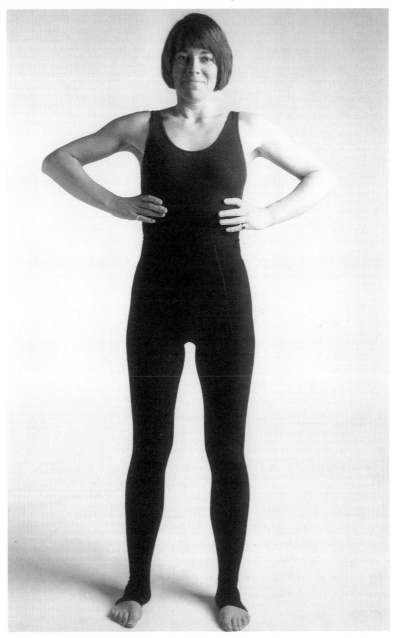

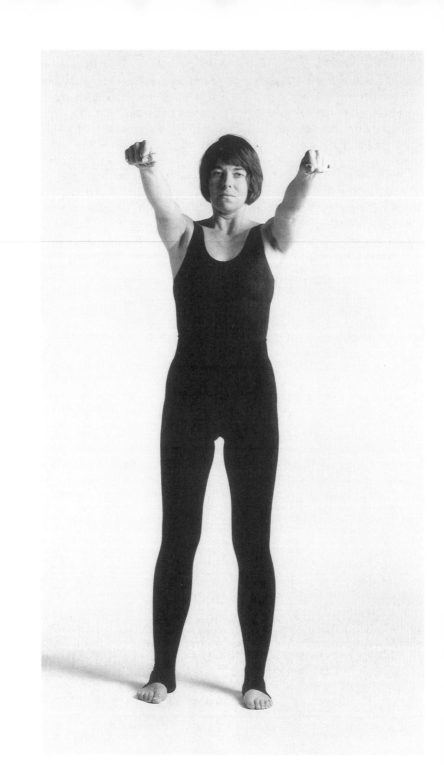

Breathing Exercise 2

This exercise is for chest expansion.

Stand erect. Inhale a complete breath and retain the air. Extend both arms forward and bring the two clenched fists together on a level with the shoulders. Then swing back the fists vigorously until the arms stand out straight sideways from the shoulders, exhaling through the mouth. Repeat six times.

Breathing Exercise 3

Now lie on the floor on your back with a telephone book under your head. Put your hands on your stomach and breathe in, making sure that your hands rise and fall with your diaphragm. You will feel your stomach rising and falling as you breathe in and out. This is correct. If you are breathing into your chest it is wrong. Do this breathing exercise twelve times.

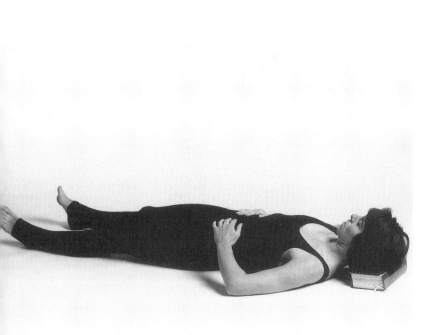

Final message from Joseph Corvo

Zone Therapy is a God-send. I believe that God has sent us Zone Therapy to help us heal ourselves, and I guarantee that 95% of all back pain can be cured simply by following the instructions in this book.

Remember that although Zone Therapy is based on sound scientific principles so that it is not just a spiritual process, there is, nevertheless, a large spiritual element involved. The power of life which keeps you alive is miraculous, and Zone Therapy is a way of using your determination and your faith to direct that miraculous power to help you achieve your goals. Believe and you will succeed.

If you want to know more about how Zone Therapy can transform your life, read my other books, ZONE THERAPY, THE NATURAL FACELIFT and THE INSTANT HEADACHE CURE. God wants you to be happy, healthy and successful. All you need is the desire to change your life and the determination to persist. Persist and the results will be miraculous.

God bless you

Joseph Corvo